EXERCISES FOR OLD FARTS

By Ned Hunter

Edited by Heidi Hunter

St. Paul, Minnesota

Exercises for Old Farts

Published by LilAbby Press
St. Paul, Minnesota
Printed in the United States of America

ISBN: 979-8-9994289-5-0 (paperback)

cover design by Heidi Hunter

graphics: Some images were generated using AI-assisted tools and edited by the editor.

DEDICATION

To all the old farts like me, who refuse to let age slow us down. May we keep moving, laughing, and living fully.

TABLE OF CONTENTS

SAFETY DISCLAIMER

The author is not a medical professional, and this book is for general fitness only. Always check with your doctor before starting a new exercise program. Stop any exercise immediately if you feel pain, dizziness, or shortness of breath. Use a stable surface for balance and wear shoes with good support.

The benefits listed with each exercise are not "all-inclusive." They will vary by individual and are included to highlight potential benefits.

INTRODUCTION

Welcome! This exercise program helps older adults ("old farts") stay active, limber, and strong, and improve their mobility. They are designed to provide full-body conditioning.

All you need is:

- a stable surface to hold onto (like a kitchen counter, wall, or the back of a chair);

- the ability to count to ten;

- the ability to stand for fifteen minutes; and

- a genuine desire to feel better and move more easily.

This program is about moving safely, stretching your muscles, and keeping your joints healthy. You don't need any fancy equipment, and you can do it in the privacy of your home.

Important Tips Before You Start

1. **Good posture is key.** Stand tall, shoulders back, head up. Remember to breathe normally as you move.

2. **Adjust the number of repetitions to your fitness level.** Ten repetitions may be plenty for someone

over 90. People in their 70s and 80s may do more. Always listen to your body.

3. **Talk to your doctor first.** Check with your doctor before starting any new exercise routine.

4. **Establish a daily routine.** Decide where, when, and how often you'll exercise. Will you exercise twice per day, or a few days per week? Morning is usually the best time to exercise.

5. **Stick to it.** Even a few enjoyable exercises every day are better than sitting still.

6. **Go slowly if needed.** These exercises are meant to limber you up. If one feels too hard, reduce the number or take a break.

Remember the motto: Exercise is the gateway to a brighter day.

Let's exercise!

Assume the Starting Position

Each exercise will begin by assuming one of the starting positions. However, you may start any exercise in this book in position #1 for added balance and stability.

Position #1

Stand tall, feet hip-width apart, hands lightly resting on a stable surface (counter, sink, wall, or chair back).

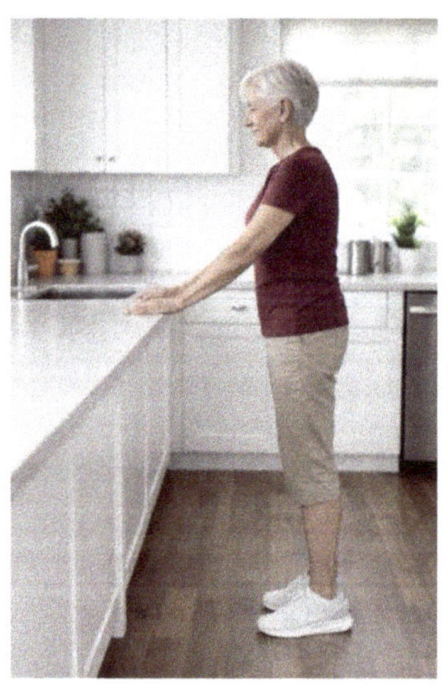

Position #2

Stand sideways (perpendicular) to the counter or wall. One hand rests lightly on the surface for balance. The other hand rests at your side. Stand tall.

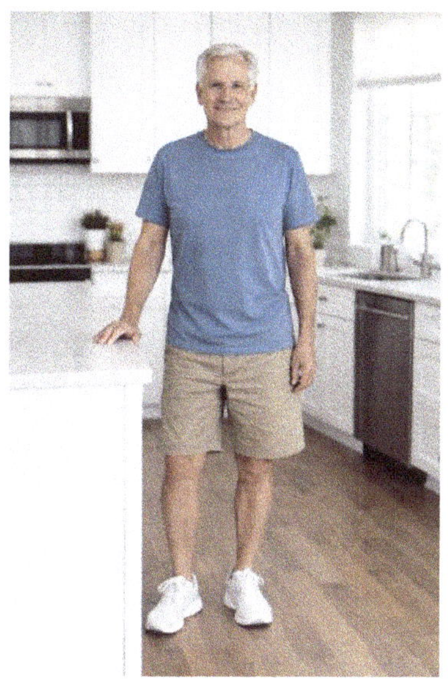

HEAD SHAKE (WARMUP)

Assume one of the starting positions.

Rotate your head slowly from side to side, looking over one shoulder, then the other as if shaking your head "no". Repeat several times.

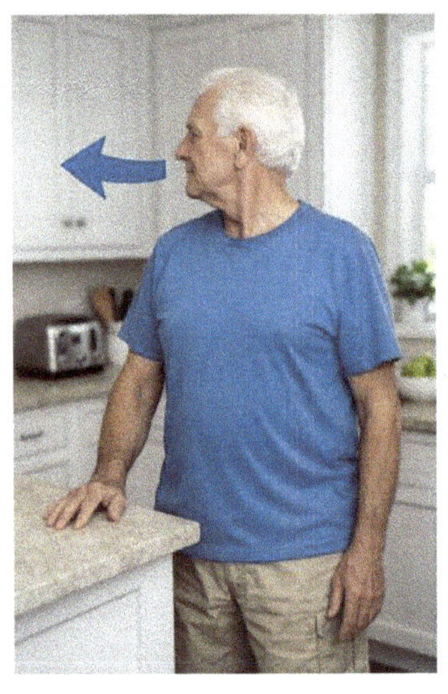 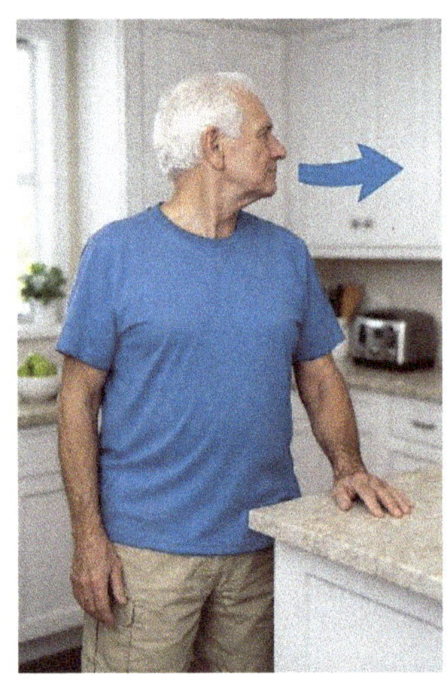

Safety tip:

Don't turn your head so far that you feel pain or discomfort.

Benefit:

Keeps your neck loose, helps you turn your head safely, and reduces stiffness.

HEAD NOD (WARM UP)

Assume one of the starting positions.

Nod your head slowly up and down as if nodding "yes". Repeat several times.

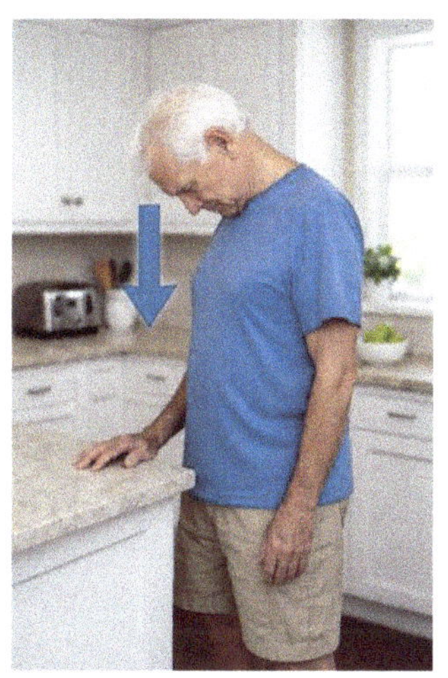 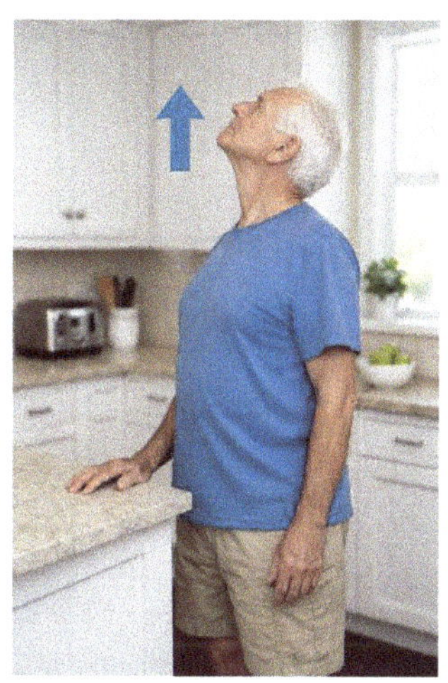

Safety tip:

Don't move your head so far that you feel pain or discomfort.

Benefits:

- Keeps your neck loose, reduces tension, improves posture, and readies your body for other exercises.
- Helps you look up and down at shelves or stairs safely.

SHAKE IT OFF (RESET EXERCISE)

After each exercise, "shake off" the body part you worked to relax the muscle worked and reset your body before starting the next exercise.

1. Gently shake your arm or leg as if you are shaking off a bug.
2. Move it in small circles, forward and back, and side to side.
3. Keep the rest of your body relaxed.
4. Breathe normally.
5. Switch sides.
6. Shake for five-ten seconds on each side.

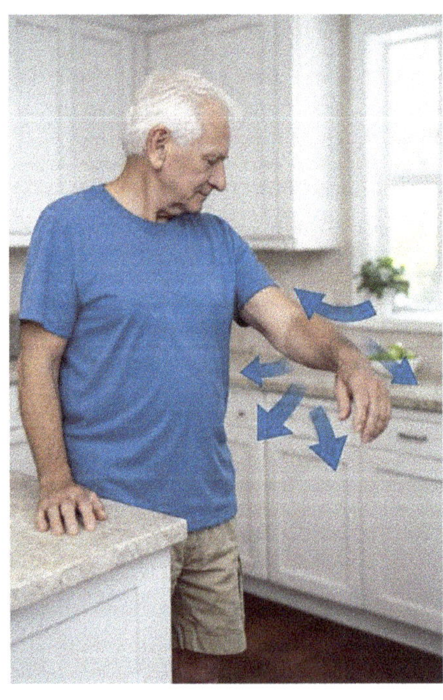

Safety Tip:

Don't shake your body part so vigorously that you feel discomfort or lose balance.

Benefit:

Loosens your muscles, improves blood flow, reduces stiffness, and helps muscles relax after exertion.

LEG SWING

Assume starting position #2, sideways to the counter, right hand on the counter, both feet on the floor.

1. Swing your left leg out to a 45° angle, then back to the starting position.

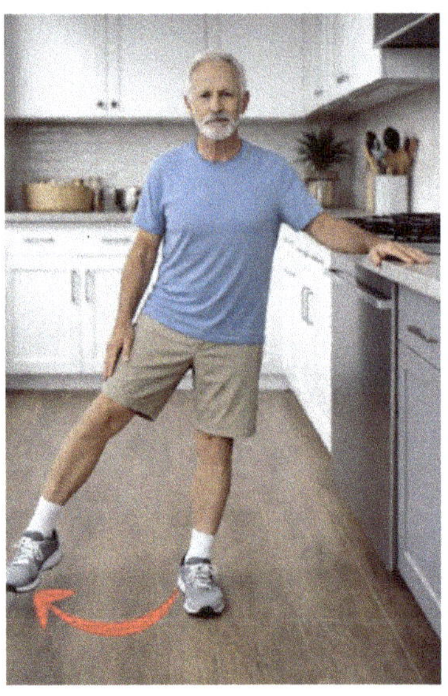

2. Do ten repetitions.

3. Switch sides, resting your left hand on the counter, and repeat with the right leg.

Safety tips:

- Keep your back straight.
- Don't swing too fast.
- Maintain balance and avoid falls by resting one hand on the counter.

Benefit:
Improves hip flexibility and strengthens the inner thigh muscles.

THE MARCH

Assume starting position #1, facing the counter, with both hands resting lightly on the counter.

1. Lift your knees one at a time, as if marching.

2. Alternate legs with each lift.

3. Do ten repetitions per leg.

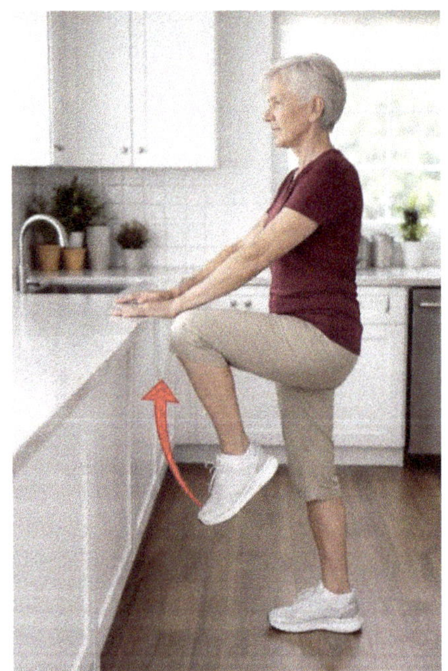

Safety tips:

- Keep your back straight and lift with control.
- Don't lift your knee higher than is comfortable. Even a small lift off the floor is effective.

Benefits:

- Loosens stiff hips.
- Helps you lift your feet more easily when walking and climbing stairs.
- Improves balance and leg control.

LEG SQUAT

Assume starting position #2 perpendicular to the counter, one hand resting lightly on the counter.

1. Bend knees to a 90° angle.

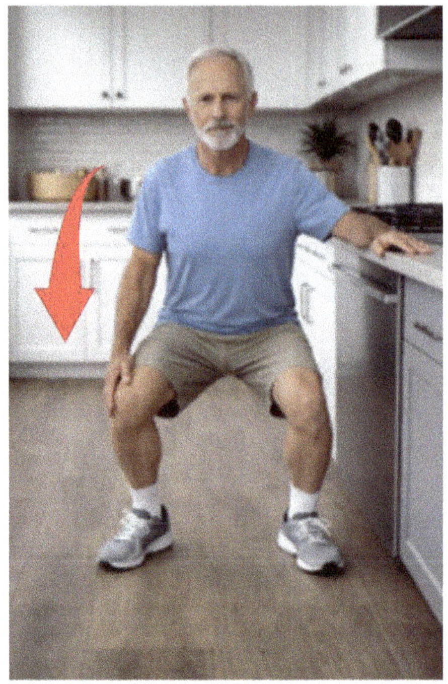

2. Stand back up to the starting position.

3. Do ten repetitions.

Safety tip: Keep your back straight as you squat. Don't lean forward.

Benefits:

- Strengthens the thighs and hips.
- Improves knee mobility.

- Improves balance.
- Makes standing up easier.
- Helps with climbing stairs.
- Supports better posture.

PUSH UPS (Counter Version)

Assume starting position #1, facing counter, both hands resting on the counter.

1. Step back about six inches so your body leans slightly forward, but your arms are still straight.

2. Bend elbows and lean toward the counter. Push back up.

3. Repeat ten times.

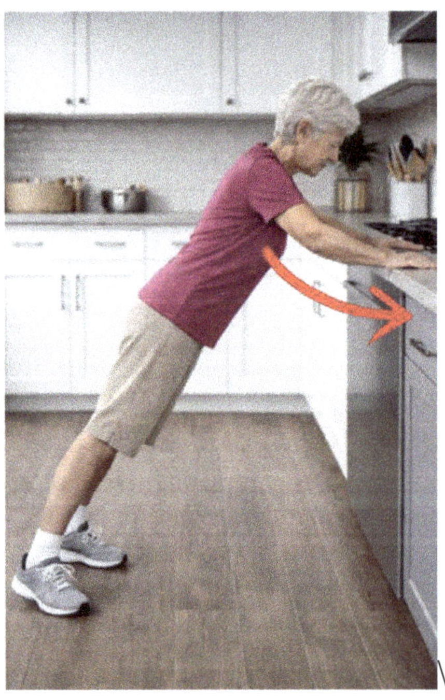

Safety tip: Keep your body straight from head to heels. Don't sag or arch your back.

Benefits:

- Strengthens the upper body - arms, shoulders, and chest—making it easier to push open heavy doors, get up from the floor, lift groceries, push yourself up from a chair or bed.
- Strengthen the muscles that support and stabilize the shoulder joint.
- Posture improvements - helps prevent rounded shoulders and encourages better upright posture.

BELLY ROLL

Assume starting position #2, perpendicular to the counter, one hand resting on the counter.

1. Rotate your midsection (abdomen) in a circle five times clockwise, then five times counterclockwise.

2. Repeat until you've completed ten belly roll circuits.

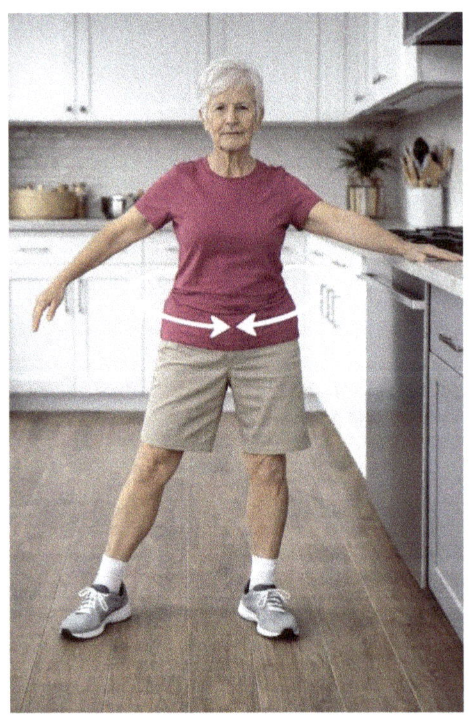

Safety tips:

- Move slowly.
- Try not make your circles so large that you feel back pain.

Benefit:

Strengthens your core to support your back and improve balance and posture.

ARM SWING

Assume starting position #2, standing perpendicular to the counter, right hand resting lightly on the counter.

1. Swing your left arm up and back down to the starting position (visualize a bird flapping its wing).

2. Do ten arm swings.

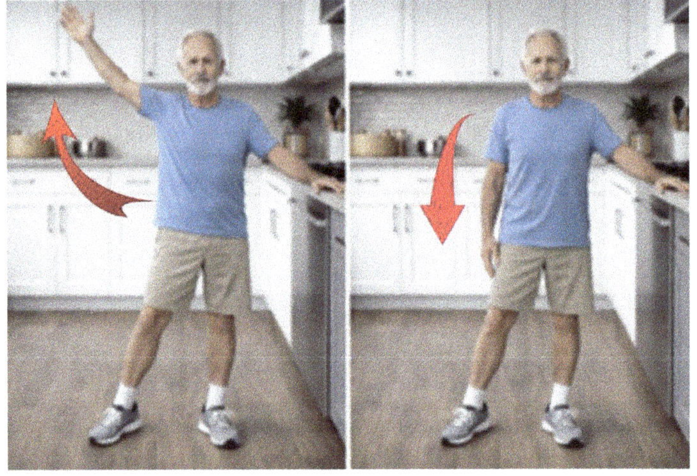

3. Turn around and rest your left hand on the counter.

4. Repeat the swing with your right arm.

Safety tip: Keep your movements controlled. Don't overextend your shoulder or lift higher than is comfortable.

Benefits:

- Increases range of motion and reduces stiffness.
- Helps shoulders move smoothly and comfortably.
- Improves arm mobility and coordination.
- Supports better balance while walking.

ARM ROLL

Assume starting position #2, standing perpendicular to the counter, right hand resting lightly on the counter.

1. Extend the left arm straight.

2. Rotate arm in small circles, palm facing up, then palm facing down.

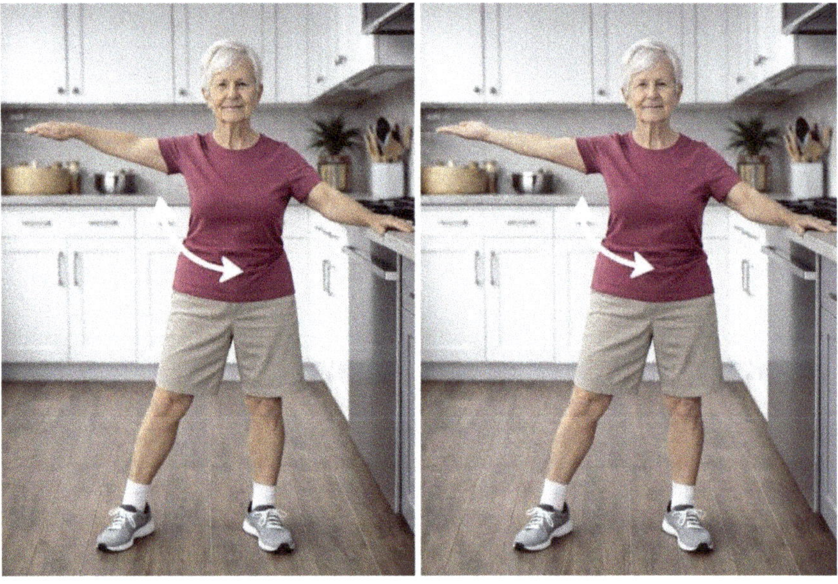

- Do ten rotations.

- Turn around and rest your left hand on the counter.

- Repeat the exercise with the right arm.

Safety tip: Move slowly and keep the movements small. Stop if you feel pain.

Benefits:

- Improves range of motion in the shoulder.
- Supports shoulder joint health.
- Improves posture.

RING THE BELL

Assume starting position #2, standing perpendicular to the counter, right hand resting lightly on the counter.

1. Bend the left arm 90 degrees at the elbow, left fist pointing up.

2. Move the left arm up and down like pulling a rope.

3. Do ten reps.

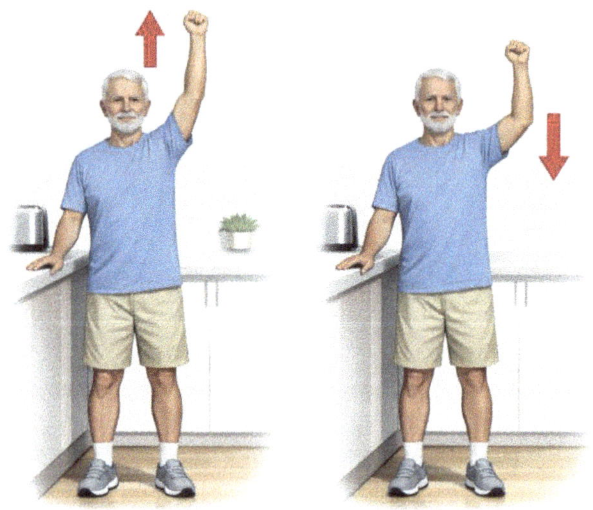

3. Turn around and rest your left hand on the counter.

4. Repeat the exercise with the right arm.

Safety tip:

- Keep your back straight.
- Don't raise your arm or shoulder too high. Use smaller movements if discomfort occurs.

Benefits:

- Improves range of motion in the shoulder.
- Supports shoulder joint health.
- Strengthens the upper body by engaging the shoulders and upper back.
- Improves posture.
- Supports activities of daily living, such as reaching into an upper cupboard and dressing.

KARATE PUNCH

Assume starting position #2, standing perpendicular to the counter, right hand resting on the counter.

1. Cock your left hand (bend at the elbow).

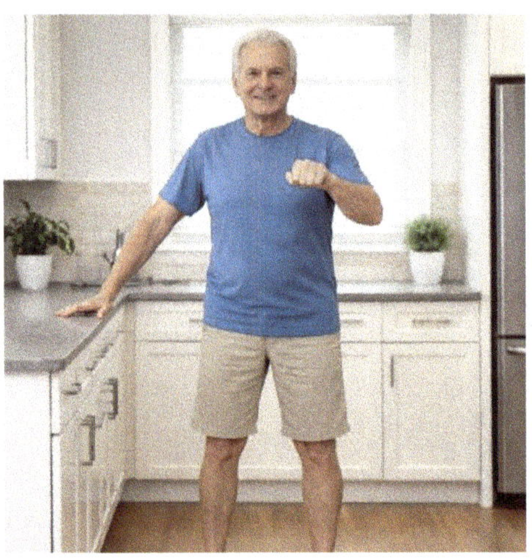

2. Punch forward at stomach level.

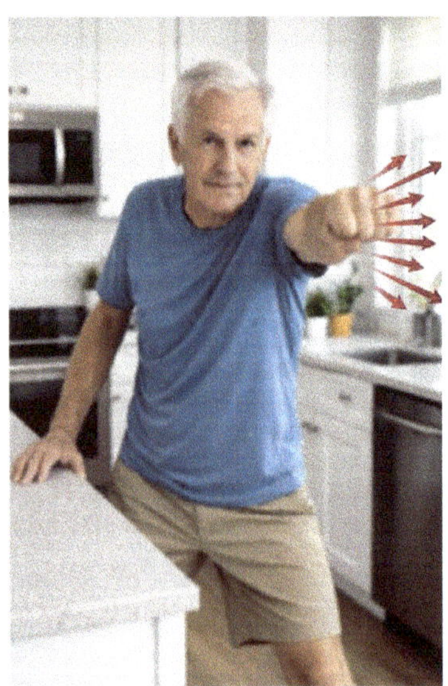

3. Pull arm back until bent.

4. Do ten punches per arm.

Safety tips:

- Move slowly.
- Don't punch too hard.
- Keep your shoulder relaxed.

Benefits:

- Strengthens the arms, shoulders, and chest, making everyday tasks like pushing, lifting, or carrying easier.
- Enhances fine motor skills.
- Activates core muscles for stability.
- Supports overall balance by helping with weight transfer and standing control.
- Improves the ability to reach, push, and interact with objects safely.

KNEE SQUAT

Assume starting position #1, facing the counter, with both hands resting on the counter.

1. Step one foot slightly forward (about six inches).

2. Bend knees slowly to squat, keeping your back straight.

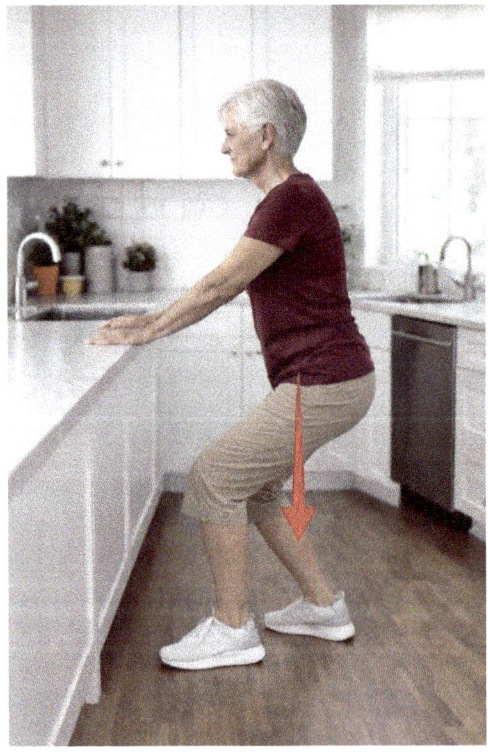

3. Return to standing.

4. Do ten squats, then switch feet so the other foot is forward.

5. Repeat ten repetitions.

Safety tip:

- Keep back straight.
- Squat straight down; don't bend forward or backward.
- Don't let knees go past toes. Keep weight on heels.

Benefits:

- Improves flexibility and range of motion in the knees and hips.
- Strengthens the thighs, glutes, and hips, which will make standing up, sitting down, and climbing stairs easier.
- Helps maintain an upright, stable posture.
- Reduces the risk of falls by improving weight transfer and lower-body control.
- Supports safe movement in everyday activities like getting out of a chair, stepping over curbs, or bending down.

HEEL LIFT

Assume starting position #2, perpendicular to the counter, with one hand resting on the counter.

1. Rise onto your toes, lifting your heels off the floor.

2. Lower heels back to the floor to the starting position.

3. Repeat ten times.

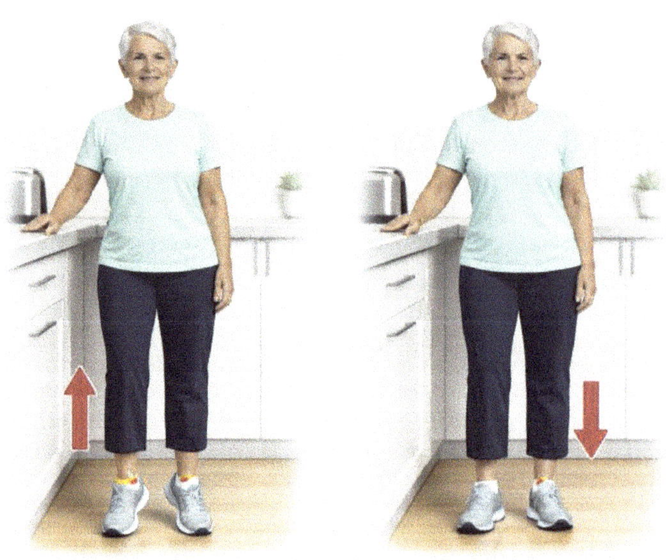

Safety tips:

- Hold the counter for balance to prevent falls.
- Make your lift smaller if you feel any discomfort in calves or toes.

Benefits:

- Builds strength in calves and thighs and improves ankle stability.
- Supports everyday movements like walking and climbing stairs.
- Helps maintain upright posture while standing.
- Reduces the risk of falls by strengthening the lower legs.
- Promotes circulation to reduce stiffness and cramping.
- Makes standing on tiptoe or reaching for high objects easier.

STEP OVER THE CAN

Assume starting position #2, perpendicular to the counter, right hand resting on the counter.

1. Place a small can on the floor right next to one foot.

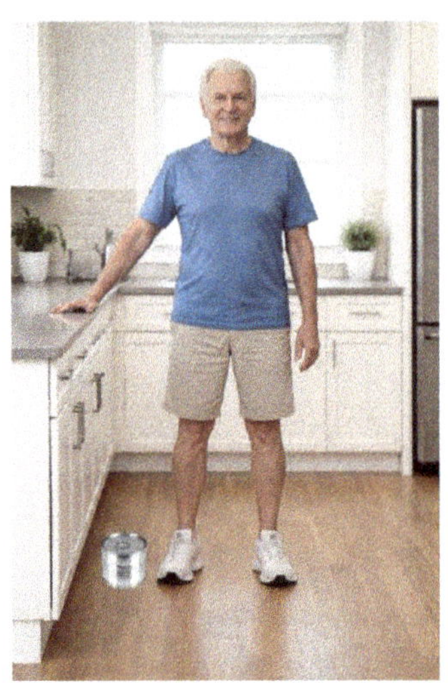

2. Lift your leg and step over the can, placing your foot down on the other side of the can so the can sits between your feet.

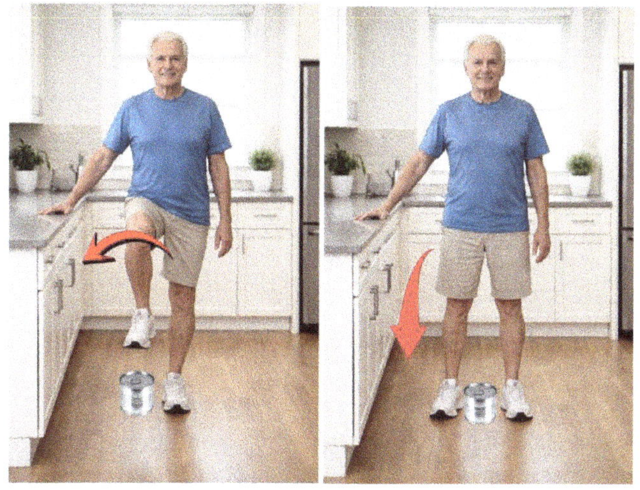

3. Lift leg and step back over the can, returning to the starting position.

4. Do ten reps.

5. Move the can to the outside of the other foot.

6. Repeat the step-over with the other foot for ten reps.

Safety tips:

- Make sure the can is sturdy and won't roll.
- Make sure the can isn't too large.
- Place the can close to your foot to maintain balance while stepping over it.
- Don't lift your leg too far to step over it so that you lose balance. A small lift will do.

Benefits:

- Improves knee and hip flexibility.
- Strengthens thighs, hips, and glutes.
- Increases balance and stability, including balancing on a single leg, weight shifting, and coordination, reducing the risk of falls.
- Helps with stepping over obstacles safely (like curbs, small objects, or door thresholds).
- Improves walking confidence and agility.
- Engages the core to maintain an upright, stable posture.

STEP BACK

Assume starting position #1, facing the counter, with both hands resting on the counter.

1. Step back with one foot about twelve to eighteen inches.

2. Then step forward, back to the starting position.

3. Next, step back with the other foot.

4. Alternate stepping back on each foot.

5. Do ten reps per leg.

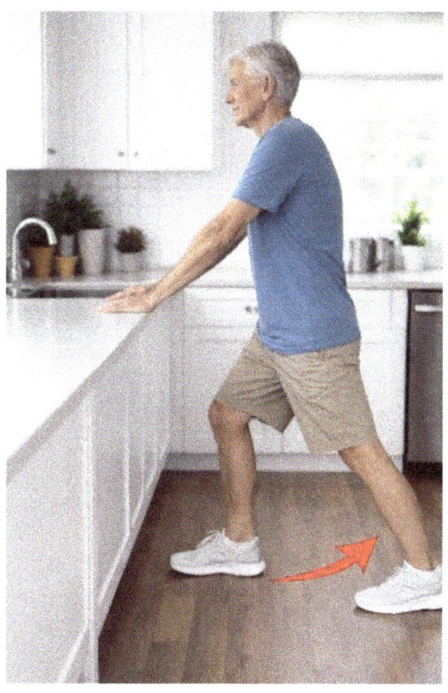

Safety tip:

- Maintain balance with both hands on the counter.
- Keep back straight and don't step back so far you're leaning forward.

Benefits:

- Builds strength in knees, calves, and thighs and improves ankle stability to support safe walking.
- Improves balance and stability by training single-leg balance, enhancing and reducing the risk of falls.
- Engages core muscles to maintain upright posture.

FINAL NOTES AND ENCOURAGEMENT

The final exercise is to give yourself a good pat on the back for a job well done!

Remember:

- Go at your own pace.
- Do these exercises daily, if possible.
- Stay safe and use support if needed.
- Don't continue an exercise if it hurts.
- Most Importantly - have fun! Moving every day keeps you limber, strong, and happy.

ABOUT THE AUTHOR

People of my age, 92, are often called "Old Farts." Usually, this label is reserved for those who are physically inactive, immobile, or infirm. I'm here to prove it doesn't have to be that way!

These exercises won't turn you into Superman or Superwoman, but they *will* improve how you approach growing older. DON'T LET AGE ROB YOU OF YOUR GOLDEN YEARS.

Designed to keep you moving, these exercises will help you make the most of your "golden years" and may even help prolong them. Whether you're just starting a fitness routine or getting back into one, this program will give you a solid start and a bit of fun along the way.